GROW & TELL

A Guide to increase Self-Worth & Self-Confidence
FOR Clinicians, Coaches and individuals: A DO-The-Work Guide

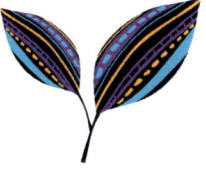

Crystal S. Brown, LMSW

Copyright © 2021 Crystal S. Brown

ALL RIGHTS RESERVED. Any unauthorized reprint or use of this material is prohibited. No part of this book may be reproduced or transmitted in any form or by any electronic or mechanical means, including photographing, recording or by any information storage and retrieval systems, without written permission from the author or the publisher, except for the use of brief quotations embodied in critical articles and review. For more information contact:

Shirley LaTour, support@slelitepublishing.com
Or Crystal Brown at www.chattinwithcrystal.com

Publisher: SL Elite Publishing
451-D East Central Texas Expy
Suite 276
Harker Heights, TX 76548

Grow and Tell may be purchased at special quantity discounts. Resale opportunities are available for donor programs, fund raising, book clubs, or other educational purposes for schools and universities. For more information contact: Shirley LaTour, support@slelitepublishing.com or slelitepublishing.com

ISBN (Paperback): 978-1-950289-40-0
ISBN (EBook): 978-1-950289-41-7

www.slelitepublishing.com

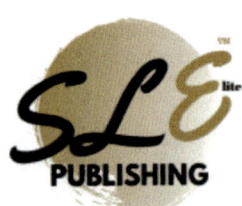

TABLE OF CONTENTS

Dedication

Intro (Conquer Your Insecurities To Gain The Confidence And Success You Deserve)

Section I
1. 10 Causes Of Low Self Esteem
2. Stages of Change fact sheet
3. 5 Surprising Ways to Develop More Confidence
4. Self-Authority: What It Really Means to Believe in Yourself
5. I Am Comfortable With My Achievements
6. I Am Admired And Respected
7. I Acknowledge My Needs
8. Enrich Your Life By Embracing Your Individuality
9. Good Self-Care Assessment
10. Taking Care Of You 6 Self Care Rituals That Soothe

Section II
11. Self-Sabotage-How-to-Banish-Self-Destructive-Behaviors
    1. Self-Sabotage Defined
    2. How Self-Sabotage Impacts Your Life
    3. Do You Self-Sabotage?
    4. Changing Your Life Strategy: Banishing Self-Sabotage
    5. Summary
12. Self-Love Means Accepting Who I Am
13. Negative-Self-Talk-Evaluation
14. My Thoughts And Actions Are Grounded In Confidence
15. My Feet Are On The Right Path
16. It Is Time For Me To Shine
17. I Have A Bright And Engaging Emotional Future
18. I Give Myself As Much Love As I Give To Others
19. I Feel Secure In My Sense Of Direction In Life
20. I Feel Free To Express Myself Openly
21. I Discover More About Myself Each Day
22. I celebrate my body
23. I am trustworthy
24. I Am Proud Of My Body
25. 8 Easy Steps to Greater Self Esteem With Affirmations
26. I Am In Control Of My Life
27. 14 Ways To Be More Loving Toward Yourself

DEDICATION

I've always wanted to be someone who changed lives in such a way that made an impact, and along the way I've learned that small achievements amount to monumental accomplishments. Putting together this book was an accomplishment that has complemented several of my previous successes. It has been most therapeutic and provided me with healing that I can only hope each of my clients, colleagues, friends and family will experience.

I would like to sincerely thank my family and friends for always being great support to me through all the challenges and celebrating with me during all the accomplishments. My father, husband, children, siblings, extended family members and closest friends: I don't have the strongest of words to express my gratitude and appreciation but know I hold the deepest love for each of you. Specifically, to my supportive husband, Chad Brown, Sr. and to my children, Sincere, Serenity, Chad Jr. and Mareena: there are not enough words in the dictionary to explain the love that I hold for each of you. You all bring insurmountable joy to my life and constantly give me reason to be motivated to be the best wife, mother and role model possible.

I would like to highlight some of my most profound successes as a wife, mother, veteran, Licensed Master's Social Worker, Life Coach, trusted family member, friend and daughter etc. With all this being said, I honor all the important statuses and I don't take any of them for granted.

I would like to recognize my mother, Lucille Gibbs-Lucas, may she sleep in peace for being such a wise, loving and great example as a mother. My love for you continues to live in my heart and I know I have made you proud.

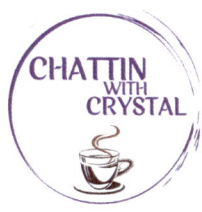

INTRO

Conquer Your Insecurities To Gain The Confidence And Success You Deserve

Our insecurities often stem from a fear of failure. This could be a good thing if you're weighing the risk versus reward of doing something that puts you in danger. But more often than not, insecurities just hold you back from having what you want in life.

Insecurities can prevent you from getting the job you want or the promotion you deserve. If you feel like you're not good enough, you may stop trying. And if you do try, the person responsible for giving you the job or promotion may pick up on your insecurities and offer the position to someone else.

If you're insecure, it can hurt your relationships as well. If you're constantly worried that your significant other is cheating on you, or is planning to leave you for someone else, this can put a lot of strain on your relationship.

A lot of individuals have financial insecurities, too. Financial insecurities can prevent you from making an investment that could be worth a lot of money in the future.

Take these steps to gain confidence and conquer your insecurities:

1. Take an objective look at yourself. Pinpoint some of the things you're insecure about and consider what you would tell someone else in the same position.

- If you're insecure about an upcoming job interview or your romantic relationship, consider what advice you'd give to someone in the same situation.

2. Stop living in fear. Maybe someone else will get the position you want. Maybe that investment won't work out and you might lose some money. Keep in mind that there's no reward without risk.

- If you let fear hold you back from trying, you'll continue to evade success.

3. Make a list of the things you're afraid of. Write down the things that make you uncomfortable and why you think they cause you to worry. Review your list and think about whether these are legitimate, rational concerns.

- Most people have a fear of failure and that's perfectly natural. However, it's important to avoid letting that fear overwhelm you to the point where it prevents you from going after the things you want.

4. Focus on past successes. Many times, insecurities stem from a traumatic experience in the past. Find a way to remember the positive experiences you've had rather than the negative.

- Maybe your girlfriend cheated on you and you're worried that it will happen again. Perhaps you had a job interview that went horribly and left you feeling defeated. Whatever the situation, it's time to move past it.

- Instead of dwelling on the times you've failed, focus on instances where you've experienced success. This will help you gain confidence and get past your insecurities.

5. Realize that you're unable to control others, but you can control yourself. It's difficult to predict the behavior of others. Your significant other may decide to break up with you and move onto another relationship. Your boss may decide that you don't deserve the promotion. None of that is within your control. You can only take ownership of your own actions.

- You can work hard to be the best boyfriend or girlfriend. You can do everything in your power to get that promotion. Focus on the things that you can control and let the cards fall where they may.

When you dwell on your insecurities, you create a self-fulfilling prophecy. You can drive people away in relationships. You could lose a job or promotion because you believe you're unworthy. Try to implement these strategies to get past your insecurities. It will give you the best chance for success.

SECTION I

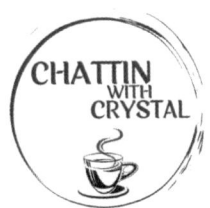

10 Factors that Contribute to Low Self-Esteem

Do you suffer from low self-esteem and wonder about the source of your feelings of inadequacy? There are many potential sources of low self-esteem. It has been said that we spend the last 60 years of life recovering from the first 18. In many cases, the first 18 years of life give our self-esteem a beating. Adults aren't immune from self-esteem issues either.

Increasing your self-esteem will enrich your life in countless ways. Your social life, finances, and happiness can all grow.

Determine the factors that contribute to your self-esteem challenges:

1. Peers. This is especially true during the school-age years, but can apply to adults as well. It's natural to want to be respected and liked by one's peers. Bullying, teasing, and other social-related issues can result in a loss of self-esteem.

2. Family. Some parents just aren't nice people. Unsupportive, critical parents or other family members can harm a child's self-esteem. This can then be carried into adulthood. If your parents were less than spectacular, remember that you're not alone.

3. Previous mistakes. Everyone makes mistakes, but some people forgive themselves more easily than others. The past is over. Look forward to new experiences.

4. Negative recurring thoughts. Negative thought patterns over years and decades can create a negative self-image. That's why it's so important to say positive things to yourself. Avoid underestimating the power of your thoughts.

5. Failure. Whether you failed to win the big game or land the big client, any perceived failure can result in a loss of confidence and self-esteem. Reframe how you view failure. Learn from your undesirable results. Only get upset with yourself if you continue to fail in the same manner. Change your approach if it isn't working.

6. Unreasonable goals. Goals that are too big lead to failure. Ensure that your goals are challenging, but within reason for you. Getting too carried away increases the likelihood of a negative outcome and poor self-esteem.

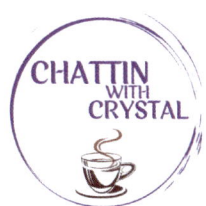

10 Factors that Contribute to Low Self-Esteem

7. Body Image. Society judges people based on appearances. You might be doing the same to yourself. Strive to move your body toward a healthy ideal but accept that everyone is shaped differently and change can take time. Females are more likely to suffer from body image issues, but males can also face challenges.

8. Trauma. Trauma can take many forms: sexual, physical, or emotional. Any of these can result in low self-esteem. If you're suffering from the results of traumatic experiences, getting professional help can be a wise decision.

9. Poor academic performance. School has a social component, but it's supposed to be about the academics. Poor grades can be viewed as failing the purpose of attending school in the first place. Ensure that your child has the academic support they need to be successful.

10. Media. Media puts forth images of success and beauty that are out of reach for the average person. It doesn't help that many of those images are manufactured and inaccurate. Holding yourself to an unreasonable standard impacts how you feel about yourself. If you must compare yourself to someone, use a reasonable frame of reference.

***Low self-esteem is a common issue. Understanding the factors that contribute to your low opinion of yourself can help to determine the solution. Everyone deals with low self-esteem days. But suffering from low self-esteem over a long period of time can lead to depression. Examine your past and find the source of your negative self-image.

Tip: Develop a plan for changing your feelings about yourself. Focus on the positive and let go of the past.

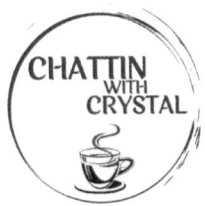

Stages of Change
FACT SHEET

Understanding where you are in the stages of change is very helpful. Take a look at the following examples. Where are you in the change process?

Precontemplation – "My doctor said I should consider hiring a personal trainer."

- At this point change is not on your radar, but you may be getting messages from others that they are concerned about some aspect of your life.

Contemplation – "I am considering hiring a trainer to help me get healthy – any recommendations?"

- You are considering making a change – gathering information, thinking about options and determining the best plan for you. This is a time of ambivalence. You are uncomfortable, but not miserable.

Determination – "I made an appointment for my first training session."

- You have decided that you want to make a change. Your situation has become uncomfortable enough to prompt change. You are committed to doing things differently. You have chosen to take the next step.

Action – "I have weekly sessions with a trainer to help with my fitness goals."

- You have taken action to change your life. You took a risk and initiated the change you want. You are doing it!

Maintenance – "My training sessions are once a month now to save money."

- This is a high-risk time for a lapse. Excitement wanes and commitment wavers. Excuses and barriers seem more difficult to overcome.

(Adapted from Changing for Good, James Prochaska)

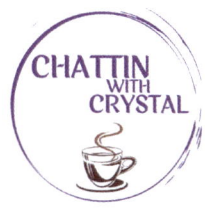

Stages of Change
FACT SHEET

Lapse/Relapse – "I haven't seen my trainer in a long time. I stopped tracking my fitness goals."

- You have stopped taking action or have begun to do it infrequently. Life seems to get complicated, and your resolve has weakened. You are off track.

Start over - "I need to call my trainer to schedule a session."

- You either begin to contemplate or convince yourself to get back on track. The sooner you move into action, the better. Remember how good it was before? You can go directly to action at any point.

(Adapted from Changing for Good, James Prochaska)

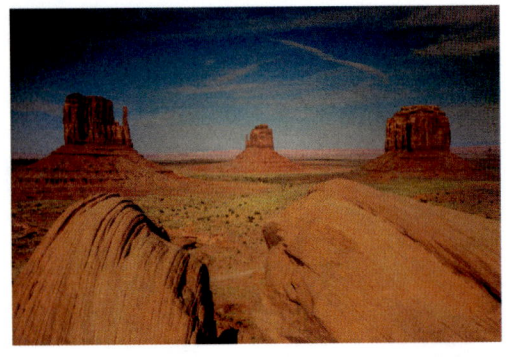

5 Surprising Ways to Develop More Confidence

We all look for a little extra confidence when we're trying to establish ourselves in our jobs, social life, or when we go out on a first date. Confidence affects our lives in many important ways.

Confidence breeds success! Whatever your goal, you're more likely to reach it if you believe in yourself.

You're more likely to seek solutions and overcome challenges because you expect positive results.

All in all, you'll get more of what you want when your confidence is backing you up.

Think about how different your life could be if you went into every situation with unlimited confidence!

Luckily, there are techniques you can practice, increasing your confidence.

Try these strategies to boost your confidence and get more of what you want, more often:

1. Be Proud of Yourself

Wherever you stand in life, it's important to be proud of yourself. Whether you're young, old, rich, or poor, you still have much to be proud of.

Chances are, you've worked hard to get to where you are today, and you deserve to be proud of everything you've accomplished. Even if you feel like you're lacking in some areas of your life, you may be rich in other areas.

Being proud of yourself will help to show others that you believe in yourself. This strength, in turn, will encourage them to believe in you, too. Their belief will serve to boost your confidence even more. It's a win-win cycle.

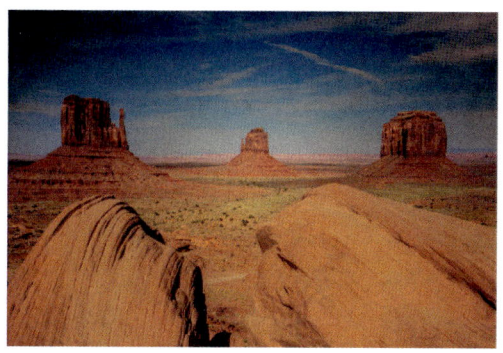

5 Surprising Ways to Develop More Confidence

2. Be Decisive

Confident people make decisions. Even if it's the wrong decision, trying out your best guess based on the circumstances will usually be better than doing nothing at all.

Once you decide, take immediate action to follow through. Others will respect your decisiveness and support you, bringing you greater confidence.

3. Ask for Help When Necessary

Being humble and asking for help is essential in developing confidence. Even the most intelligent people the world has seen have asked for help when it was needed.

Not only will this help you to feel more confident in your decisions, but it can also help you to develop stronger relationships.

4. Do Something Difficult Everyday

Constantly challenging yourself can be one of the best things you can do for your personal confidence level.

Taking on difficult tasks will help to challenge you in ways that you wouldn't consider inside your comfort zone. But, leaving your comfort zone to achieve something - anything - can show you strengths and talents that you never even realized that you had.

5. Help Others Whenever Possible

When you help someone else, you benefit, too. However you choose to help, it makes you feel more capable. You feel good about yourself for helping because you had the resources, skills, or funds to help them.

Helping others will also give you practice in new ways of communicating and make you more outgoing as you reach out to extend a helping hand.
Developing greater confidence is certainly a worthwhile goal! It will make you more successful in every facet of your life.

Self-Authority: What It Really Means to Believe in Yourself

Nobody but you can be the final authority on your life. If you don't step up in that role, someone else will try to fill it for you. Empower yourself to stake a claim over your own life.

The phrase, "Believe in yourself," is a common piece of advice. But, what does it really mean? Although part of it is self-confidence, there's a deeper meaning to be found and appreciated.

Believing in yourself is about self-awareness

Deep down, you know what you're able and unable to do. When you believe in yourself, others are unable to pressure you into doing anything you don't want to do. On the other hand, no one can hold you back from doing something you know you can do.

Outside perspective is important, but nobody knows you like you know yourself. With regular introspection, you can build unshakable self-confidence. The Delphic maxim "Know thyself," inscribed for all posterity on the Temple of Apollo, speaks to this truth.

What are your strengths? What are your weaknesses? Only you can answer these questions. You're the only person in the world who truly knows your capabilities. Too often, people walk away from opportunities muttering "coulda," "woulda," "shoulda."

The Importance of Self-Esteem

Self-esteem needs to be cultivated, just like a garden. Weeds, in the form of negative self-talk, can creep in at any time.

High self-esteem can help you communicate better, make you more decisive, earn you the respect of others, and allow you to maintain your integrity.

Increasing your self-esteem becomes an exercise in writing a self-fulfilling prophecy. As you build your confidence, you'll empower yourself to achieve more in your personal and professional life.

Believe in Yourself

Some think of self-doubt as a monster, greedily sucking away their motivation. This outlook isn't particularly helpful because it sends signals to the subconscious that can strengthen self-doubt even more. Instead, be aware that self-doubt is a part of you that's vulnerable and in need of support.

Take these steps and increase your self-esteem starting now:

1. Explore self-doubt. Doubt is part of the human experience, just like joy, fear, and sorrow.

If you discover what's at the root of self-doubt and explore that, you may find that the doubt loosens its paralyzing grip. This will help you stop fighting with yourself, and you can move toward your goals.

The key is to get to the bottom of your insecurities and face your fears. Addressing your fears is easier if you itemize them first. Putting your fears down on paper puts them in perspective.

2. Take stock of your fears. Your fears will appear menacing when they're staring at you from within your own mental space.

Record your fears daily, in a journal, and watch the list shrink before your eyes.

3. Pay attention to your thoughts. Another way that you can cultivate self-confidence is to listen to your internal dialog.
Your fears can lurk in the words you use to describe yourself. Instead of saying, "I won't be good at this," try, "How can I make myself better?" out for size. Powered by TCPDF (www.tcpdf.org)

Consider separating yourself from chronically negative people. Cutting ties with toxic people is difficult but do what's best for you. Becoming assertive will allow you to help yourself and others.

4. Relish your successes but avoid living in the past. When you're feeling down, it's easy to focus on your failures. Instead, recall your past successes. It's okay to feel grateful for all that you have.

Maintaining an optimistic mindset will help you recognize opportunities when they arise.

Ultimately, believing in yourself means claiming self-authority. Avoid letting others make decisions for you or limit your potential. Often, these people are projecting their own self-doubts onto you. Focus on your goals and talents and remember you deserve success.

I Am Comfortable with My Achievements

I am at peace with my achievements. I avoid comparisons to the achievements of others. I am happy with what I accomplish every day.

I am grateful to have a list of accomplishments in my mind. My achievements show my progress over time. They reveal how I grow as a person and how my soul changes with each new experience.

My previous achievements motivate me to do more.

My past lets me see how to make my present and future even better. My accomplishments show me a successful path.

I am comfortable with what I do and what I achieve. I understand my efforts matter in every way. I avoid negative thoughts that force me to judge my accomplishments against the achievements of others.

I am modest and humble, yet I am comfortable sharing my achievements. I avoid boasts that make others feel uncomfortable.

I am happy with my level of skills, talents, education, and background.

Today, I am comfortable with my accomplishments and avoid the pain that comes with comparisons or critiques. I know my achievements are unique and are part of my individual life path. My accomplishments help my friends and family understand the work and effort in my life.

Self-Reflection Questions:

1. How can I avoid comparing my accomplishments to what others my age admire?

2. What can I do to balance my accomplishments with my struggles?

3. How can I help family and friends understand that accolades are just one part of the human experience?

I Am Admired and Respected

I live my life according to my values. This is one of the reasons why others admire and respect me. Living by a code gives me credibility. It also makes my attitudes and behaviors understandable to others.

When others trust me, it is easier for them to respect me, too.

I have great respect for everyone I meet. Each person is unique and interesting to me. When I am willing to give respect to others, they respect me, too.

I am a good and loyal friend. I take all my relationships seriously. I make time for my family and friends. They admire me and view me positively because of the emphasis I place on my relationships with others.

I have meaningful goals that I pursue with enthusiasm. I receive admiration from others when I share my important goals.

Everyone respects those that act with purpose. I know my purpose and live it each day. I enjoy my life and share that joy with others.

I strive to be at my best each and every day. I approach each day with enthusiasm and look forward to what the day will bring. Others admire and respect my attitude.

Today, I am making an extra effort to be a shining example to the world. I keep my values in the front of my mind. I strengthen my relationships. I strive to be someone that people admire and respect.

Self-Reflection Questions:

1. Whom do I admire and respect? Why?

2. What can I do to be more worthy of admiration and respect?

3. What are my values?

4. How can I be more consistent in living my values?

I Acknowledge My Needs

I have needs just like everyone else in the world. To deny that my needs exist is to deny myself happiness. I am able to admit that I have needs.

Some view having needs as a weakness. But the willingness to express my needs shows strength. I have the courage to be honest about my needs.

By letting others know what I need, I am far more likely to have my needs satisfied. There are many people that care about me and want to see my wishes met.

I take a self-inventory to assess my needs.

By doing this, I get a better understanding of myself. I am able to set goals that put me on the path to fulfillment.

I strive to have a reserve of everything that fills my needs. I know that if I have an excess of money, love, time, and fun, my life will be immeasurably enjoyable. When my needs are unfulfilled, my life is more challenging.

When I have everything I need, I am at my most capable.

Enrich Your Life By Embracing Your Individuality

Do you find it difficult to accept the person you are? Maybe you feel discomfort about being so different from everyone else. Or perhaps you find yourself similar to others to the point that you believe you're boring.

Either way, it's time to recognize that your special variety of character traits combine to create a one and only, unique you.

Although there are many ways to accept and embrace who you are, check out these strategies to open your arms to the amazing individual you are:

1. Take note of your habits. What kind of habits do you practice? Do you floss your teeth every night and consistently wash dishes as soon as you dirty them? Is your bedtime and time for arising always the same?

Understand what's important to you by noticing the behaviors you routinely do. In a sense, your habits are your "trademark."

2. Describe your personality in detail. A wonderful technique for embracing your individuality is to think deeply about the type of person you are. If you had to describe yourself to another human being, what words would you use?

Maybe you're always in a hurry or like to keep a very clean house. Perhaps you have a lot of friends and are quite gregarious.

Write down your description of yourself and be as thoughtful and thorough about your personality characteristics as you can. You're worth the time this strategy will take.

3. What is so great about you? Of course, you have your own special blend of positive qualities, like being a good listener, having a good sense of humor, and being dependable for others.

4. Identify your biggest struggles. What challenges you? If you're ever stumped about how to handle a situation, describe those situations on paper. Getting a handle on what taxes you the most increases your self-awareness.

5. Work to improve how you handle your biggest struggles. Yes, identification is great but tackling each challenge one by one to experience success in those areas is very important to do for yourself. Why? Because you'll see that you can overcome anything you set your mind to. Delve into self-improvement to learn more about the unique person you are.

6. Remind yourself that you're a decent human being. In order to embrace your individuality, you must accept who you are. Learning to love yourself and take yourself as you are is a great aid to loving and encouraging others. Sure, you have flaws, but who doesn't?

Keep in mind that recognizing you're okay doesn't mean you can't or shouldn't work to improve. In fact, accepting your foibles and less-than-perfect characteristics can help you improve.

7. Vow to embrace who you are each morning. It's a new day. You have opportunities to experience discoveries about yourself and who you are. Consider the unfolding day as a venue to keep learning more and more about yourself.

Actively work each day to love your individuality. Notice your habits. Stay in close touch with the elements of your personality. Know what is great about you as well as what kinds of things vex you.

*** Embracing your individuality and accepting yourself for exactly who you are will enrich your life in ways you can't imagine. ***

Good Self-Care Assessment

Rate each statement with one of the following:

1 – Rarely   2 – Sometimes   3 – Frequently

___ I get plenty of rest and sleep 7-8 hours daily.

___ I eat healthy foods and regular meals.

___ I maintain contact with people who support me emotionally.

___ I exercise 30 minutes or more 3-5 times per week.

___ I take a break at work every 1 – 1.5 hours to stretch and move around.

___ I engage in spiritual activities regularly.

___ I play! I do something fun at least once a week.

___ I nurture my relationships – call/write/email/visit/talk/date.

___ I get outside daily – the fresh air and lush greenery are good for me!

___ I use my down time to rejuvenate – do something I enjoy.

Scoring:
Review your responses and consider the following for each statement.

1 – Rarely   Needs improvement - let's talk about how to strengthen this area.
2 – Sometimes   Good job! We can come up with ideas to help you be more consistent.
3 – Frequently   Great job! Keep up the good work!

Taking Care of You: 6 Self-Care Rituals That Soothe

Most of us can't deny that life gets way too busy. So busy, sometimes, that you may feel like you don't have time to take care of yourself. In order to embrace all that life has to offer, move self-care to the top of your list.

The rituals you practice taking care of your mind, body and soul can be soothing and contribute to the contentment and joy you feel in everything you do.

Review these self-care rituals to remind yourself how important you are. Then, revive some of your own practices or add new ones that soothe you.

1. **Practice soothing, healthful skin care. Regardless of whether you're a man or a woman, your skin needs all the help it can get. After all, skin protects you 24/7.**

Morning and evening, clean, tone and moisturize your face.

Apply lotion to your body at least once a day to protect your skin from excessive dryness.

2. **Exercise. Exercising relieves your stress and rejuvenates both your mind and body.**
Even if you just exercise 15 minutes twice a day (morning and evening), getting the physical activity your body craves will revive your mood and enrich your life profoundly.

Try a 10-minute walk to give your mind a rest or lift your spirits. Whether you choose a brisk pace or a slow saunter to admire the landscape, consider it a gift to yourself to go for a brief stroll.

3. **Re-acquaint yourself with the magic and exhilaration that nature provides.**

Nothing relaxes and nurtures us like getting outdoors.

Find time to sit on your porch to watch the birds.

Take a few minutes to care for a flower garden or go for a walk in the park.

Taking Care of You: 6 Self-Care Rituals That Soothe

4. **Shower daily. Bathing is one of the top self-soothing moments of your day. By adjusting one or two things about your shower, it becomes a relaxing ritual you can look forward to.**

Rather than rush through your bath or shower every morning and evening, take the time to soothe yourself by using a luscious soap or that new loofah sponge or bath puff.

Light scented candles, put on relaxing music, and take the time to fully enjoy them.

5. **Take time to do the one thing you really love to do. There's something so delightful and special about having the time and space to do whatever it is that you get excited about.**

Maybe you've got an insatiable love of reading, but struggle to find the time to read with working and family tasks tugging at you. Or perhaps you like to sew or work with wood. No matter what your beloved activity, figure out a way to make it happen.

Even if it's every other day or once a week, an important part of self-care is doing what makes your heart sing.

6. **Stay in touch with your feelings. You may think this sounds somewhat cliché. But the truth is that if you're honest with yourself about how you feel, you'll have more peace and contentment inside.**

Living your life based on your real feelings will bring comfort and joy to your soul. It can be a challenge to be truthful with yourself and others about how you feel. But if you do, the rewards are great.

Engaging in activities and rituals that soothe you deep inside enriches your day-to-day existence. A regular practice of self-care also demonstrates that you truly recognize your own worth. Discover a deeply satisfying life through practicing soul-soothing, self-care rituals.

SELF SABOTAGE

HOW TO BANISH SELF DESTRUCTIVE BEHAVIORS

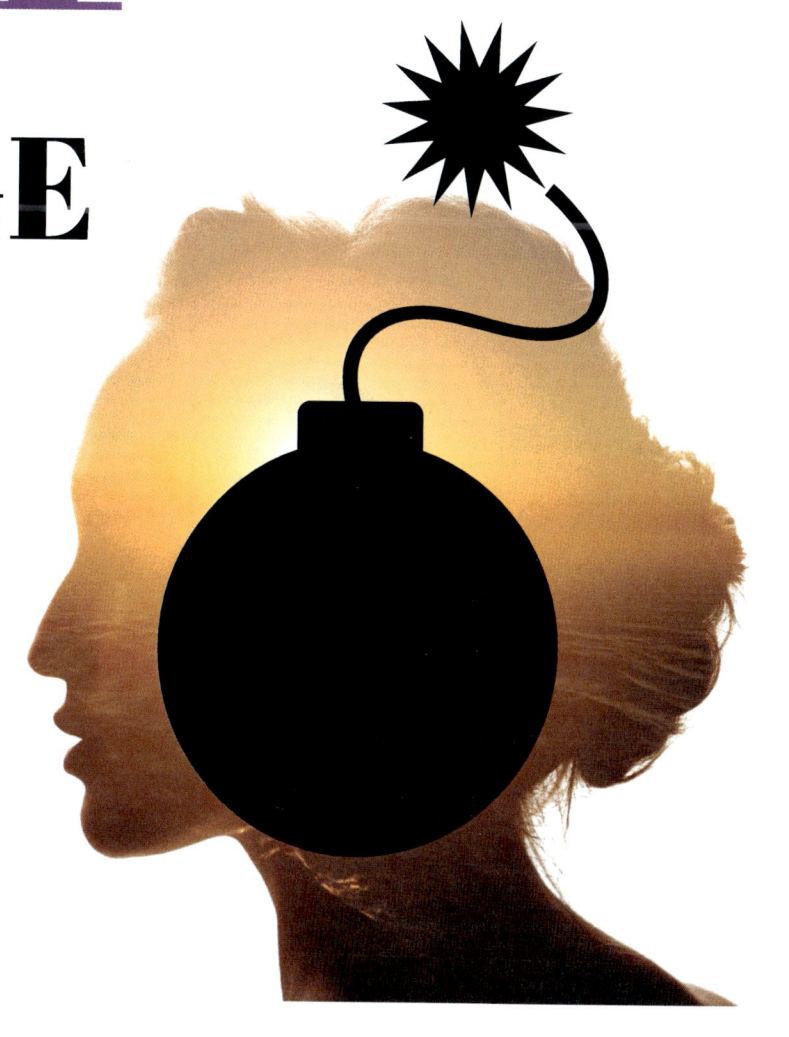

SECTION II

Self-Sabotage Defined

How Self-Sabotage Impacts Your Life

Do You Self-Sabotage?

Changing Your Life Strategy: Banishing Self-Sabotage

Summary

> "I have never been contained except I made the prison."
> – Mary Evans

Self-sabotage, while seemingly easy to define, can be made up of a complex set of actions. If you've ever found yourself interfering with the positive parts of your own life, you've experienced this intricate set of thoughts, feelings, and behaviors. But don't worry... you can unlearn these habits today!

This book defines self-sabotage and explains how you may be defeating yourself and keeping yourself from reaching your goals. In case you're still not sure whether you engage in these behaviors, the impact of self-sabotage on your life is also discussed.

But best of all, this book details easy steps to help you banish self-destructive behaviors for good! By using these strategies, you can live the more satisfied and successful life you so richly deserve.

Self-Sabotage Defined

Self-sabotage involves engaging in behaviors that lead to results you don't want. Maybe you've heard the old expression, "shooting yourself in the foot." If so, then you understand the concept of self-defeating behaviors.

When you do something that ultimately hurts or thwarts you in some way, you engage in self-sabotage. By performing these destructive actions, you are bringing negative experiences and situations into your life.

However, self-sabotage is complicated because there's usually some element of temporary relief, short-term payoff, or avoidance of something negative initially in the process.

Unfortunately, these brief episodes of positive feelings only serve to reinforce the idea that there are benefits from engaging in the problematic behavior.

To further muddle the picture, you'll eventually begin to feel the negative longer-term results of your questionable behavioral choices. So even though there's an early payoff, you'll ultimately get stung when you engage in self-defeating actions. Although self-sabotage is quite common, your efforts to avoid performing these types of troublesome behaviors will be worth your while.

The process of self-sabotage usually begins in your thoughts and feelings. Then, you make a choice based on those ideas and emotions.

Here's an example of self-sabotage:

You've been going to the gym for several months, but then you went on holiday, skipped going to the gym for a few weeks, and gained 15 pounds.

You're embarrassed and you don't want anyone to see you like this, so you choose to stop going to the gym entirely. That way, no one will see you've gained weight, and nobody will see you in your now ill-fitting workout clothes.

The immediate consequence of your choice is that you don't have to risk being stared at by the others at the gym. You won't have to even momentarily experience the humiliation you feel about your weight, particularly in front of people you perceive as thin and dedicated to their health.

You feel a bit relieved. You think, "I'm so glad I don't have to deal with the whole health club thing." However, the ultimate result of your decision not to go to the gym is that you hold on to the extra 15 pounds or put on even more weight. Is this what you were hoping for?

Obviously, those results are opposite what you wanted when you joined the gym. The decision to skip exercising and avoid your feelings of discomfort only compounded your challenges in losing weight. This decision exemplifies self-sabotage; not only do you not get what you want, but you get more of what you don't want!

> "Self-sabotage is when we say we want something and then go about making sure it doesn't happen."
> - Alyce P. Cornyn-Selby

How Self-Sabotage Impacts Your Life

As you might surmise, self-sabotage can drastically affect your life. Self-defeating behaviors will most likely bring unfortunate circumstances your way.

Check out these important points about how self-sabotage reduces your quality of life and results in unplanned consequences:

1. Self-sabotage becomes easier over time. When you choose to practice self-sabotage, your choices become easier to repeat. You may fall into a habit of doing whatever is necessary to avoid initial uncomfortable feelings, thoughts, and situations.

2. Self-defeating behaviors cause unintended consequences. Unfortunately, there are long-term results of your choices and behaviors that you might not expect and therefore are unprepared for. Like in the example above, often the long-term effects are the exact opposite of what you originally wanted.

3. Any positive results of self-sabotage are short-term. Remember that any seeming benefits you experience due to self-defeating decisions aren't long-lived. Some examples of short-term positive results are:

- You get out of giving a short speech to the supervisors at work so you won't feel anxious. Although this may seem like a great benefit, you lose your opportunity to practice speaking in front of others, which could reduce your anxiety next time. Instead, now you have reinforced the idea that you are too scared to speak to a group.

- You initially feel better about not being chosen to complete a big project at work: no stress! Plus, you won't have to do as much work as your co-workers at the moment. The long-term consequences of this can be diverse, but one of the biggest effects is that you have less opportunity to practice working under pressure. Therefore, you don't get better at it.

- You choose to stay with your abusive partner; therefore you don't have to pack up and find a place to live. Clearly, the long-term results of this choice can be dire, regardless of how much stress it may alleviate in the short-term.

- You won't have to sweat it out in an uncomfortable job interview since you didn't apply for the position. What? You're okay with only applying for jobs that you know you can get? You don't want to advance your career? The long-term results of this choice can lead to lower income over your lifetime, reduced self-esteem, and less job satisfaction.

- You keep hanging out with familiar people even though they aren't very positive. After all, it's easier than making new friends. This one can affect everything in your life. We become like the people we spend the most time around, so if you want to be happy with your life, affiliate with happy people!

4. Regular self-sabotage drastically alters your life. The scariest aspect of self-sabotage is that if you make it a habit, in several years' time (or less!), you may find yourself not living the life you truly want. In fact, you'll likely experience great difficulty accomplishing the goals that you've set for yourself. Essentially, you'll stop believing in yourself.

Self-sabotage occurs over all periods of time, from minutes to years. Although you might experience a brief period of feeling better after an incident of self-defeating behavior, as time goes by, you're bound to experience unpleasant consequences.

> "The haft of the arrow had been feathered with one of the eagle's own Lures. We often give our enemies the means of our own destruction."
>
> – Aesop

Do You Self-Sabotage?

The nature of self-defeating behaviors is that they tend to be pervasive in the lives of people who engage in them.

If you self-sabotage sometimes, you probably self-sabotage much of the time. This becomes your primary way of thinking, choosing, and relating. Self-sabotage comes in many forms.

These examples show how you might be practicing self-sabotage:

1. Drinking too much alcohol at social events. If you drink a bit more when you're going to be around new people, you may help yourself relax a bit and be a better conversationalist. However, don't be surprised if you occasionally make a fool of yourself instead.

▸ A function of drinking too much is a reduction in your good judgment. Isn't that the last thing you want if you're hoping to meet new people and make new friends?

2. Saying "yes" when you'd like to say "no." Agreeing to do extra tasks when you have no real desire (or time) to do them is a classic way to self-sabotage.

‣In fact, if you end up not getting something done when you agreed to do it, your friends and family will be disappointed, annoyed, or even angry with you. Most likely, these were not the results you were looking for when you said "yes" to the task!

3. Insisting on your own way. Many of us do this out of a desire to seem knowledgeable and capable. But how do you suppose people feel about you if you refuse to cooperate and, instead, must have things your way? Do they respect you or see you as a person of knowledge and wisdom?

‣If your goal is to be respected and taken seriously, you're self-sabotaging if you insist on having your own way all the time.

4. Reacting instead of responding. Acting out your feelings isn't always best. Sometimes, you need to take a step back and evaluate the situation before you act.

‣For example, perhaps you feel anxious, so you avoid doing something, even though you know that you ought to follow through. Or perhaps you feel angry about something a colleague said. Self-defeating behavior in this case might include lashing out at them, which would just cause further friction in your relationship.

5. Believing and behaving as if you're always right. Deep down, if you feel you "must" be right and others must be wrong, you probably lack true confidence. Otherwise, you wouldn't care what others thought.

‣When you behave this way, you destroy your relationships with others. And that's most likely very contrary to your true goal.

6. Refusing to take care of your body. How can you work hard, enjoy the love of others, and live a healthy, fulfilling life if you don't take steps to take care of yourself? Regular exercise is required for all. Ignoring that fact is a refusal on your part to do all that you can for yourself and your body, which is indisputably self-defeating.

7. Maintaining an unhealthy diet. Consistently eating poorly isn't healthy, whether you're skipping your fruits and vegetables or taking in too many calories.

‣Probably the most common self-defeating behavior in the U.S. is knowingly overeating and consuming high fat, low-nutrition foods. It's self-sabotage in its purest form.

8. Avoiding things you don't want to do. Whether the object of your avoidance makes you anxious or you think it requires too much work, refusing to participate in some things can sabotage your efforts to have a fulfilling and successful life.

9. Taking a passive stance to avoid a fight. Perhaps there are times when your feelings matter but instead, you just keep your thoughts and emotions to yourself so you don't rock the boat. Later, though, you end up in a swamp of difficulties because of initially holding in your honest responses.

10. Procrastinating. Even though you tell yourself you want to do something, you just keep putting it off. Before you know it, you've missed the deadline or you're still in the same position you didn't want to be in.

The short-term payoff may be more time for other things initially, but the long-term results always include increased stress.

11. Not finishing what you've started. Whether it's that painting you started that's been in your closet for years, the scrapbook from your last vacation, or the bookshelves you were making out in the garage, perhaps you have a habit of not finishing things.

Eventually, you become frustrated from all your unfinished projects.

12. Being indecisive. Perhaps you just let time go by without deciding about something important in your life.

You believe you're escaping the stress of making the decision when, in fact, you're letting a wonderful opportunity go by. This is how people miss their opportunities to marry someone they love or get that new job they've been dreaming about.

13. Avoiding getting a handle on your finances. You've convinced yourself your finances are out of your control. This way, you don't have to make any efforts to correct them. You simply blame it on your boss or the economy. This self-sabotage costs you money and a more secure lifestyle.

14. Taking a pessimistic approach to life. When you consistently focus on the negative aspects of your existence, you vastly limit your choices in life. A negative perspective means you simply won't see certain options. You'll be stuck in a never-ending cycle of pessimism.

15. Non-suicidal self-injury. In its most extreme form, self-sabotage can be physically unhealthy and even dangerous. Non-suicidal self-injury, NSSI, is a newer term for self-injurious behaviors, like cutting yourself, sticking pins in your skin, or burning yourself intentionally with matches or lighters.

▸Although those who engage in NSSI have reasons, such as stress or depression, these behaviors usually have the unintended consequences of embarrassment, avoidance of others, and social isolation.

The range of human self-destructive behaviors is wide and deep. There are a multitude of methods you might be engaging in, including self-defeating thinking, choices, and actions. Contemplate your own thoughts and decisions to determine if you're taking part in any self-sabotaging behaviors.

> "This is how women self-sabotage and self-destruct. Unless we have constant witnesses to our hard work, we are convinced we pull off every day of our lives through smoke and mirrors."
>
> – Sarah Breathnach

Changing Your Life Strategy: Banishing Self-Sabotage

Although letting go of your self-sabotaging behaviors isn't always easy, you can succeed if you make it a priority. Thankfully, there's a full range of strategies you can employ to help yourself avoid self-sabotaging behaviors.

To start your journey of eliminating self-destructive behaviors, commit to follow these steps:

1. Acknowledge that you engage in self-sabotage. Just like the first step in Alcoholics Anonymous, it's important to admit to yourself that you have a challenge before you can do anything to change it.

2.   Write out how you self-sabotage. This exercise will feel like you're cleaning out the clutter of a closet, only it's your mind and emotions you're sorting through instead. Keep thinking and writing until you've listed all the ways you engage in self-defeating behaviors.

▸Next, put down specific incidents where you recognize that your thoughts, choices, or behaviors were self-defeating. Go back for at least the last year or two.

3.   Claim full responsibility for your thoughts and actions. Now is the time to step up and do whatever is necessary to let go of the self-defeating thinking and behavior. Own it.

4.   Plan your responses to challenging situations. Write them down! For each of your episodes of self-sabotage you wrote down in Step 2, record how you'll respond in a similar situation from today forward. Be specific.

▸For example:

"I will not avoid going out with friends just because someone I've never met will be there. Instead, I'll go with them and make an effort to talk to the new person. It's okay if I feel some anxiety! I won't allow my tense feelings to push me toward a decision that will ultimately prevent me from making new friends, which is important to me."

5.   Share your plans with a close friend or family member. Let someone know what you're working on. This part is important: ask them to confront you whenever they see you engaging in any self-sabotaging behavior. If you choose someone you trust, you'll believe them when they tell you you're self-sabotaging.

▸If your friend comes to you to share that you're about to self-sabotage, carefully consider the information. Then thank them for telling you and ask them to continue to follow through with letting you know in the future about such behaviors.

6.   Tell yourself you're worth the effort. Those who fall into repeated patterns of self-sabotage have low self-esteem and simply don't feel worthy of experiencing the lives they want. This is no secret.

Repeat to yourself that you're worth the time and effort to change your self-defeating thinking and behavior.

7.   Get out of the rut: start believing in yourself. Rather than put yourself down, give yourself some props for making it this far and for recognizing your self-defeating ways.

Keep reminding yourself that you're letting go of the old style of living where you lacked confidence and determination. Make a decision to believe in yourself again.

8.   Make a vow to yourself and a close friend. Commit to working to decrease, and eventually stop, engaging in self-sabotage. Say it out loud, to yourself and to your friend. If it helps you, feel free to say it to yourself in front of your bathroom mirror.

9.   Use thought-stopping techniques to end unhelpful thinking. Negative thoughts can lead to self-sabotage. Whenever unproductive thinking begins, imagine a big red light in your mind, blocking out the negative ideas. Then, imagine a green light while choosing to replace the negative cognition with a positive one.

▸For example, let's say you're trying to eat healthier. As soon as you begin thinking about eating doughnuts, visualize a big red light. Then, think about eating an apple instead. Visualize a green light as you get the apple and bite into its crunchy sweetness.

10.   Give yourself positive reinforcement. Making changes can be challenging. Using the example in Step 4, remind yourself during your evening with new friends that you made the right choice to get to know more people. Give yourself a mental pat on the back. You're going for your goals. Good for you!

11.   Acknowledge your new, positive feelings and experiences. Staying with the example in Step 4, maybe you met three new people or made a real friend. Perhaps you laughed all evening and really had a great time. You might have even gained some confidence regarding socializing with new people.

▸As you begin to make different choices, you'll notice a pronounced drop in the number of your self-sabotaging actions. Bask in the positive emotions you feel about making healthier choices.

12.   Educate yourself. Read a variety of self-improvement books about feelings to be better informed about what goes on inside of you.

Engaging in self-study enriches your life in many ways and will help you re-focus your efforts on what you truly want.

Here are some examples:

- *Feeling Good: The New Mood Therapy* by David Burns.
- *The Book of Awakening: Having the Life You Want by Being Present to the Life You Have* by Mark Nepo.
- *Change Your Thoughts - Change Your Life: Living the Wisdom of the Tao* by Dr. Wayne W. Dyer

Don't limit yourself to these though!

There are abundant options in the self-help section of your local bookstore and more are written all the time.

If you find some that appeal to you more than the titles above, read them instead. This is all about self-discovery, and that starts with tuning in to what you really want!

13. Keep your eyes open. Vigilantly monitor your thoughts and emotions. Notice when those self-destructive ideas creep into your mind. Stay in touch with your feelings. This way, you'll have greater awareness and can evaluate emotions and thoughts before they become behaviors.

14. Give yourself permission to think outside the box. Be willing to let new and foreign ideas into your head. Allow yourself to engage in new ways of thinking.

15. Consider professional help. If you don't feel like you're able to decrease your self-sabotaging behaviors, consider seeking professional assistance. Therapists, social workers, life coaches, and mental health counselors will help you confront your unhealthy thoughts and behaviors and develop effective ways of dealing with them.

- Many people seek professional assistance at some point in their lives and doing so can benefit just about anyone.

16. Persevere. Although there may be times when you feel overwhelmed by your ability to self-sabotage and contemplate giving up, if you persevere, your life will get better. Look back over these steps often. Re-read what you wrote about the ways you self-sabotage and how you'll overcome it.

- As you practice these steps, you'll discover new ways to approach your challenges. You'll find that you possess greater strength and courage. One day, you'll look back and notice that you've come farther than you ever imagined possible. That day is worth all the challenges between here and there.

17. *Renew your commitment to yourself as often as needed.* When making a commitment, all of us occasionally veer off-track. When you notice this, make a new commitment to yourself to continue in your endeavors to banish self-sabotage.

To do away with self-defeat for good, place these 17 steps on your refrigerator or by your bedside table where you'll see them every day. Review them often. Once or twice a day is a good place to start. Take time to think about what you're doing in your efforts to end your self-sabotage.

Keep your wish to banish self-destructive acts in the forefront of your mind. Your awareness is critical to your recovery.

> "My definition of a mistake is when you don't follow your rules. And if you don't have rules, then everything you do is a mistake. And self-sabotage occurs when you keep repeating the same mistakes over and over and over again."
> – Van K. Tharp

Summary of Self Sabotage

Self-sabotage involves a complicated set of circumstances that ultimately short-circuits your ability to meet your goals.

Repeated episodes of self-defeating behaviors will have devastating effects. And the ways you might be self-sabotaging are diverse. Most of us engage in this in some form, and for many of us, it pervades our lives.

However, today we've begun the path toward banishing self-destructive behaviors. Free yourself from self-sabotage to achieve your goals and live the life you've planned for yourself!

> "People who bite the hand that feeds them usually lick the boot that kicks them."
>
> – Eric Hoffer

Self-love means accepting who I am.

Beneath my exterior is a soul that deserves to be honored. It forms the essence of my being and is meant to be treated with respect. Self-love means accepting who I am on the inside. The perspective of the outside world is irrelevant.

When I achieve a sincere love for the person who I am on the inside, positive self-talk occurs naturally. Building self-love happens from the inside out.

Becoming worthy of love starts with having a character of integrity. I ensure that each of my interactions with others is handled openly and honestly. I am trustworthy and proud to be a person who speaks from the heart.

My honesty inspires others to put their trust in me. Knowing that I am a safe place for others gives me a good feeling about myself.

I also approach others with kindness, regardless of the relationship we share. Leading with kindness makes room for peaceful resolution and effective collaboration. I promote positivity.

Although I have flaws, my positive traits far exceed anything that I sometimes feel insecure about. I celebrate my strengths and embrace my imperfections. There is so much about me that is lovable.

Today, I am exactly the person who I am supposed to be, and I love every ounce of my being. There is power in truly accepting myself just the way I am. With confidence, I go through each day conquering big challenges and feeling proud of my victories.

Self-Reflection Questions:

1. What are some of my favorite personality traits?
2. How do I rebuild my confidence when I am made to feel unloved by another person?
3. What are some positive affirmations that I can repeat to myself each day?

Navigate self-talk evaluation

Check all that apply:

☐ I criticize my looks.

☐ I have negative thoughts about my best efforts.

☐ I talk myself out of trying new things.

☐ When I receive positive feedback, I say or think 'Yes, but...'

☐ I would never talk to other people the way I talk to myself.

☐ I label myself with derogatory names, such as loser, stupid, klutz, etc.

☐ When I have good thoughts, my critical inner-voice reminds me of past failures.

☐ When entering a room, I anticipate the worst.

☐ I find myself repeating the same negative thoughts automatically.

☐ I find fault with my accomplishments.

Scoring

Count the check marks.

0 – 3   **Your self talk could be better.**
4 & Above   **Let's discuss your responses.**

My thoughts and actions are grounded in confidence.

I have faith in myself and in my abilities. When I am grounded in confidence, I have positive and confident thoughts that result in positive and confident actions.

It is much more challenging to be successful or happy without confidence. On the other hand, with confidence, everything is possible.

When I lack confidence, luck plays a greater role in my future. **I can live a life free from the need for luck by being confident in myself.** I have confidence so I can have control over my thoughts, actions, and life.

My confidence is grounded in my experiences. I have many successes and I remind myself of those successes daily. My work and dedication lead to feeling more confident. My past provides the foundation for my confidence. I quickly forget any negative experiences.

If I catch myself having a thought that lacks confidence, I immediately stop and remind myself of my successes. **I only allow confident thoughts to remain in my mind.** All other thoughts are banished.

I start each day by allowing confidence to well up inside of me. It feels as if I am filled with a pure, white light. The resulting warmth gives me confidence and courage.

Today, I remind myself of my many past successes. I only entertain thoughts and actions grounded in confidence. I have faith in my abilities and intelligence.

Self-Reflection Questions:

1. What are my greatest successes so far?
2. What other things have I done that I can be proud of?
3. What are the situations that create doubt within me? What can I do to let go of that doubt?

My feet are on the right path.

I know I am on the right path for my future. I sense that happiness and fulfillment are within my reach. My feet guide me as I arrive at my full potential. I am capable of amazing things and accomplishments.

I have the ability to see the path in front of me.

I am excited about my future and work. I am overwhelmed with gratitude for the path that inspires me.

My life is an adventure!

I do work and activities that fulfill me. I enjoy the stops along my path because each one provides a learning opportunity. I appreciate the chance to see things in a different way and gain knowledge from my errors.

I have fun along my path. I share my joy with friends and family along the way.

I know obstacles are part of the path. I understand how to overcome them and move beyond them. I appreciate the opportunity to learn from these challenges.

I use my imagination as I move through the path.

I use my heart and mind to see things along the path. I watch my steps, but I also allow for the freedom to have excitement.

Today, I notice my feet are on the path to enlightenment. I am thrilled to be on this path.

Self-Reflection Questions:

1. How can I ensure I stay on the right path for my best life?
2. What can I do to avoid feeling disappointed by obstacles in my path?
3. Who can I turn to for inspiration and help along my path?

> # It is time for me to shine.

After all of these years of pretending to be smaller than I really am, it is my time to shine. **I am ready to put my best foot forward and show the world what I have to offer.**

I am tired of limiting myself. I deserve to be free and to be noticed.

I am sharing my greatest skills, talents, and gifts with the world. I am comfortable showing the world my true self. I am making my true nature available to everyone. I am sharing the best parts of myself.

I may have been too self-conscious in the past to have enough comfort to show myself to the world, but that time has passed. **Today is a new day and a new chapter in my life.**

I am growing so much that I feel like I might explode! The time has come to allow myself to be seen as I truly am.

It is my time to shine.

I am looking forward to this new lifestyle. I am open and free. I embrace my strengths and weaknesses. **I feel comfortable letting others into my life.** I am excited at the prospect of showing the world what I can do.

Today, I am willing to openly be myself. I am putting my best out into the world and accepting all the consequences, positive and negative. I am looking forward to the peace I can enjoy from taking this bold step.

Self-Reflection Questions:

1. What parts of myself am I hiding from the world? Why?

2. What will I gain if I allow myself to shine? What will I lose?

3. What do I have to offer to the world that I haven't yet?

I have a bright and engaging emotional future.

My future is bright and beautiful. I am the ruler of my emotions and I direct them toward fulfillment, peace, and joy.

As I examine my emotions, I see the beauty in them. They all have value and worth. They lead me through a happy and enjoyable experience of life every day.

Each day, I see that I can choose the direction my future takes. I make the choice to move my life forward. Emotions are an important part of my life, and I can choose how to control them. By seeing the value of my emotions, I have more understanding.

My past challenges are gone, and I let go of the emotions from them. I allow only positive thoughts and emotions into my life. Each day, I work to remove negativity so I can have joyous experiences in my life.

Others want the joy and happiness I have. They like to be around me. They find my joy refreshing and they look for more joy in their own life because of me. I love to share my bright and engaging future with others. I look for ways to advance my life.

There is always something valuable I can learn. Then, I teach that valuable information to others. Because I help others visualize their bright futures, my future looks bright as well. I look forward to what my emotional future will bring me.

Today, I see that my emotional future is bright, and it brings me great joy.

Self-Reflection Questions:

1. What can I do to keep moving forward emotionally?
2. How can I let go of any past hurts that I'm still holding onto?
3. What is the best way to show others how to embrace their emotional future?

I give myself as much love as I give to others.

I love and support my family and friends unconditionally. I celebrate their joys and lift them up during hard times. I give them the foundation they deserve.

I know I deserve the same amount of love and support that I give to my loved ones. I am continually kind to myself because I am worth it. I avoid selling myself short when it comes to appreciating who I am and what I can accomplish.

When I make a mistake, I can admit it without beating myself up about it. I analyze where I went wrong and trust that I can avoid the same error the next time.

I take the time to treat myself to nice things, just like I do with others. My treats to them represent how much I love them. When I treat myself, I feel the same kind of love.

I feel reassured when I say kind words to myself in the mirror. Even when I notice my shortcomings, I recognize that there is far more to love than to see as lacking. I choose to focus on the positive things.

There is a lot about me that makes me special. I embrace those things every day and find peace with who I am.

Today, I commit to treating myself as kindly as I treat those I love, because I love and accept myself just the way I am.

Self-Reflection Questions:

1. How can I promote greater feelings of self-love and acceptance within me?

2. Do I acknowledge my input when I contribute to a meaningful accomplishment?

3. How do I encourage myself to be positive when I feel unmotivated?

I feel secure in my sense of direction in life.

I know where I am going with my life. My greatest dreams are revealed to me again and again. I cannot hide from them, nor would I want to. I am in touch with my intuitive self, and because of this I feel secure in my sense of direction in life.

My hopes and dreams guide me. Sometimes I may need to take detours for a while, or do some foundational work so that I can get back on the primary path toward my goals. Always, I am moving forward in ways that work for me.

If I ever feel like I may be off course, I do a quick reality check.

First, I look for signs inside of me: how do I feel about the direction I am headed? If my emotions are negative, which direction elicits positive emotions when I contemplate it?

Then, I look around me: are external signs pointing me in a different direction?

If I find that my internal and external signs are both guiding me in a way other than the one that I am taking, I go with the new direction.

My ability to adapt to change and see things in new ways is an enormous boon in choosing my direction in life. These abilities help me feel secure that I am making good choices for me.

Today, I am confident that my life is going in the right direction for me. I am capable of accomplishing my dreams, so I head toward them without reservations. Each day, I make progress toward my goals, and this contributes to my security in my sense of direction.

Self-Reflection Questions:

1. In what recent situations have I felt most confident in my sense of direction in life?

2. In what circumstances have I felt unsure of myself?

3. What can I do in future situations like these to boost my self-confidence?

I feel free to express myself openly.

One of my greatest gifts is my ability to express myself openly. Although many find it challenging, I find that it is easy to let others know my thoughts and ideas.

I have many great friendships because of my openness. People trust me and find me interesting. My openness serves as an inspiration to them. It helps them see how comfortable communicating can be.

It is liberating to be free of a need to censor myself. The best parts of me are free to come out. Freely communicating my thoughts and feelings allows others to get to know the "real" me and strengthens our bonds of love or friendship.

Being able to express myself openly is an exciting way to live. It is also very peaceful. I carry this feeling of peace everywhere I go, like a suit of armor.

When I feel myself becoming self-conscious, I remember that I only have to impress myself. I know I am worthy of others' attention and have positive things to say. I can be confident that what I have to say will be received well.

Today, I feel comfortable sharing my thoughts, feelings, and ideas. People are drawn to me because of this. I am comfortable in my own skin. I show others they can be comfortable, too.

Self-Reflection Questions:

1. How much freedom do I feel to be open with people?

2. In what situations do I feel stifled or constricted?

3. What can I do to express myself more openly?

I discover more about myself each day.

Like everyone else, I am a complex and multifaceted individual. I currently enjoy many talents and gifts, but I have many more that lie untapped. I look forward to discovering all that I have to offer the world and myself.

I frequently surprise myself with my vast capabilities. This phenomenon keeps me enthusiastic. Yet, I remain humble. As I realize my own gifts, I recognize the numerous gifts that everyone else has to offer. I am more open to discovering new talents in myself if I remain humble and open-minded.

I know I have many perspectives and preferences of which I am unaware. I find myself interesting. I want to know more.

I am able to laugh at myself as I discover my quirks. These silly characteristics make me unique and lovable. I smile at myself every day.

I try new things and introduce myself to new people on a regular basis. New activities and people create opportunities to discover more about myself.

I like to reflect on how much I have grown over the years. I am encouraged to continue growing and evolving. It excites me to consider what I might experience. I wonder how powerful I can become.

Today, I look forward to discovering more about myself. I want to experience something new today and use that to unlock a new talent. I am committed to learning more about who I am.

Self-Reflection Questions:

1. What do you know about yourself today that you did not five (5) years ago?

2. What new activity would you most like to experience?

3. Do you need to add some new people to your life to fully grow into the person you could become?

I celebrate my body.

I am beautiful inside and out. I celebrate my body and work at keeping it strong and healthy.

I appreciate the things my body can do. My body keeps me alive and allows me to enjoy my daily activities. I thank my body for the opportunity to raise my family, do meaningful work, and put my faith into action.

I treat my body with love and respect.

I eat nutritious foods and stay hydrated. I fill my plate with vegetables and fruits. I prepare delicious meals and snacks at home so I can control what I put into my body. I drink water instead of sugary soft drinks or excessive alcohol.

I work out and manage my weight. I participate in my favorite sports and exercises. I follow a sensible diet I can stick with for life. I pursue realistic goals based on my body type and health needs.

I get adequate sleep and rest. I go to bed and wake up on a consistent schedule that helps me to feel refreshed and restored each morning.
I take care of my appearance. I focus on my positive qualities.

I build a network of support. I speak out when I witness fat shaming or other inappropriate behavior. Helping others to like their bodies teaches me to appreciate my own.

Today, I feel happy and comfortable in my own skin. I avoid comparing myself to others and love my body just the way it is.

Self-Reflection Questions:

1. How does my media consumption affect the way I think about my body?

2. What is one thing I like about my body?

3. What does a positive body image mean to me?

I am trustworthy.

My daily mantra is to be sincere and honest with each person I encounter. Painting an accurate picture to them brings peace of mind to both of us.

I appreciate when another person is straightforward with me so I take the same approach with them. My commitment to sincerity shows that I am easy to trust.

Close friends confide in me with their deepest secrets. When someone asks for my advice and confidence, it is easy for me to give it. I keep in mind that the treatment I expect from others is what I am obliged to give to them.

Being the custodian of another person's private details is an honor for me. I feel like it is my duty to protect them at all costs.

It is important to live with integrity because it aligns with my moral compass. Being good and honest to others is the honorable thing to do. Telling the truth is crucial to my life as a trustworthy individual. It assures me that I am able to live with a clean conscience.

Today, I present myself to those around me as a person worthy of trust. Each opportunity I get to adequately care for what is given to me is precious. The profoundness of my life is rooted in how I choose to live with those around me.

Self-Reflection Questions:

1. What do I do to gain the trust of others?

2. How do I regain the trust of someone who believes I have broken it

3. In which instances am I cautious about giving all the details to someone who asks?

I am proud of my body.

I have a positive relationship with my body - therefore I can live in my physical self with joy. I am thankful for all the many things I can accomplish in the physical world each day. I am proud of my body and all that it does for me.

My eyes allow me to read a novel, textbook, or favorite magazine. My fingers help me button my clothes, pick up a pencil to write, or find what I am looking for in a desk drawer. My voice conveys my thoughts and intentions to the world, and my ears hear what is said in return. And my brain powers all of this.

What a marvelous machine my body is!

I am always able to love my body. My weight may fluctuate. My memories may come and go. Wrinkles may form on my skin as a natural product of aging. But my body has served me all the days of my life and it continues to do so today. For this, I am grateful and proud of my body.

When I have a heavy package to lift, my body is there for me. If I cannot pick up the item by myself, my brain helps me find assistance. And if I try anyway, and feel pain, I feel grateful and proud of my body for letting me know when enough is enough!

Today, I am thankful for all my body does for me.

I feel confident in the physical world, and, although my abilities may change over time, my body always lets me know what it can and cannot do. I am proud of my body every single day.

Self-Reflection Questions:

1. What are some things I do well physically each day?
2. How does my body let me know when it has had enough?
3. How can I continue to increase my pride in my body?

8 Easy Steps to Greater Self-Esteem with Affirmations

Don't feel 100% great about yourself? Join the club. Most of us could use a little boost regarding our opinions of ourselves. Affirmations can be an effective way to boost your self-esteem.

The key to using affirmations is to state them in the positive and to use them religiously. It can take thousands of repetitions to make a dent in your current level of self-esteem.

Use this process to harness the power of affirmations to enhance your self-esteem:

1. Determine the weak areas of your self-esteem. In what aspects of your life do you feel negatively about yourself? It might be related to work or your relationships. Hone in on the areas of your self-esteem that need the most work.

2. Create affirmations that address your areas of weakness. Suppose your self-esteem regarding your work is less than you'd like. Be kind to yourself and create powerful affirmations even if they seem over the top. For example:

- I am the most capable person on my team at work.

- I contribute regularly and in a meaningful way toward solving the biggest problems at work.

- I am the person most likely to receive a promotion and a raise.

- I am calm, cool, and collected in even the most stressful work situations.

- Try to come up with a minimum of 10-15 affirmations. Make them positive and in the present tense.

3. Create an audio recording of all your affirmations. This will be used later. Ensure that the quality of the recording is decent. You don't want the sound of a phone ringing or a dog barking in the background. Your recording doesn't have to be professional quality but give it your best effort.

- Read each affirmation at a normal speaking pace and speak clearly. Leave a short pause between each affirmation.

4. Write or type each affirmation clearly on a piece of paper. It's important to be able to carry your affirmations with you everywhere. That could mean putting them on a small piece of paper or having an electronic version on your phone or tablet. Whatever format works for you is fine.

5. Spend some time each day listening to your affirmations. Ideally, at a minimum, you'll listen to them while you're lying in bed in the morning and in bed at night. Put on your headphones and listen to your affirmations repeat over and over. If you can fall asleep with your affirmations in your ear, great!

- You could even take a walk at lunchtime and listen.

6. Spend some time writing your affirmations each day. Pull out a pen and some paper and write them by hand. Typing doesn't count. This is a highly effective way of implanting your affirmations into your subconscious. It's not enjoyable, so you'll have to be tough and ensure you get it done.

7. Read your affirmations. You've been listening and writing. Now, it's time to read them. Pull out your list of affirmations and read over them a few times each day. Let your subconscious know that you're serious. Keep at it.

8. Consider a little electronic help. There are free programs you can get for your computer that will flash your affirmations on your computer screen for short periods of time. You can program them to flash for periods of time so short that you can't possibly see them consciously, but your subconscious mind will see them.

- Imagine seeing your affirmations all day long at work!

Affirmations can be a useful tool for increasing your level of self-esteem. With more self-esteem, life will be more enjoyable, and you'll be more capable. Create a few affirmations and use them several times each day. Write them, listen to them, and read them. Your self-esteem will grow.

I am in control of my life.

I have power over the direction of my life. I call the shots and make the decisions. My life is my responsibility and mine alone.

I accept the awesome responsibility of managing my life and creating the future I desire.

Regardless of my past, I have the ability to change the direction of my life. I know that I can live the life of my dreams.

I am free to make decisions that support my goals and values. I may sometimes feel that my options are limited, but that is just an illusion. I always have more options than I realize.

I am open to all the possibilities my life holds. I examine all of my available choices and make wise decisions.

I may have allowed other people to control my life in the past, but that time is over. I am firmly in control of my life now. I enjoy the power I have to steer my life in a direction that pleases me. I am free of the influence of temporary circumstances.

I have the ability to overcome significant obstacles.

Today, I exercise the power of choice and take full control of my life. Each day, I make positive decisions that can affect various aspects of my life and take responsibility for those decisions.

I am the master of my life and my future.

Self-Reflection Questions:

1. In what ways have I given up control over my life? Why?
2. What would I do if I believed I would not fail?
3. What can I do to take more control over my life each day?

14 Ways to Be More Loving Toward Yourself

What would your life be like if you treated yourself like a dear friend? After all, your attitude towards yourself shapes your daily reality.

When you're kind to yourself, you have more strength and resilience to deal with difficult times. You may even find yourself attracting more affection from others when you love yourself wholeheartedly. Accepting yourself brings you closer to discovering your inner beauty and sharing it with the world.

Pursue your own passions instead of comparing yourself to others or blindly following external expectations.

Study these 14 ways to help you let go of judgments and value yourself more.

Taking Care of Yourself:

1. Eat healthy. Self-care is one aspect of loving yourself, and following a balanced diet is fundamental. Get most of your calories from nutritious whole foods including vegetables, fruits, whole grains, lean proteins, and healthy fats.

2. Exercise regularly. Work out at least 3 days a week to strengthen your heart and muscles and increase your balance and flexibility. Incorporate more physical activity into your day by biking to work or doing chores manually.

3. Sleep well. Give your body adequate sleep and rest. Go to bed at the same time each night and invest in ergonomic bedding that supports proper posture.

4. Schedule playtime. Take a break from being serious. Playing board games or sharing a laugh helps you to engage with others and stay mentally sharp.

5. Change your self-talk. Do you speak harshly to yourself? Switch to words and messages that will encourage and inspire you.

6. Stay connected. Surround yourself with supportive family and friends. Eat dinner together as a family so you can share wholesome meals and pleasant conversation. Arrange weekly dates with friends for coffee or lunch.

7. Ask for help. Reach out for assistance when you need it. Let others know what they can do to help you resolve any challenging situation. Relationships are about give and take.

Believing in Yourself:

1. Build trust. Follow through on the promises you make to yourself and know that you can deal with life's ups and downs. Have faith in your talents and strengths.

2. Practice forgiveness. Pardon yourself and others for past disappointments. Acknowledge that each of us messes up sometimes. Look at mistakes as opportunities to learn and grow instead of beating up on yourself.

3. Set goals. Give yourself something to work towards. Design goals that are challenging and realistic. Write them down and share them with others to increase your sense of accountability. Well-defined goals can motivate you to achieve more.

Other Tips for Loving Yourself:

1. Be authentic. Take satisfaction in being true to yourself. Welcome feedback from others but trust your instincts and make your own decisions.

2. Develop gratitude. Being thankful makes you happier and boosts your self-esteem. Keep a gratitude journal or meditate on the positive aspects of your life. Express your appreciation to others by letting them know how much their kindness means to you and use it to motivate you to act generously too.

3. Do meaningful work. Spend your time on activities that align with your values and purpose in life. Think about what you find most fulfilling about your job. You might also find gratification in hobbies, volunteering, or other areas apart from your career.

4. Ask spiritual questions. While you're nurturing your body and mind, pay attention to your spirituality as well. Your faith can provide a strong foundation for understanding and loving yourself.

Make your relationship with yourself a top priority. Take care of your needs and show yourself the same love and respect you would have for anyone you cherish.

ABOUT THE AUTHOR

Who is Crystal S. Brown?

First and foremost, she is the daughter of the most high God. She is also an author, Nephrology Social Worker, Life Coach and Founder of Chattin' with Crystal, an Army Veteran, Wife, and Mother of four (4).

Currently, she is a Nephrology Social Worker, which is a social worker who works with individuals on dialysis. She enjoys working with clients in this health-care setting and assisting with increasing the quality of their life. As a social worker, she uses a strengths perspective approach to ensure that her clients are trying to live; because, without dialysis, they would die.

Mrs. Brown, LMSW is also a Life Coach and founder of Chattin' with Crystal. Life coaching is her glow up! Life Coaching is a caveat to Social Work, allowing her to work with healthy individuals who are seeking to enhance the quality of their life. She is honored to work with people who are already thriving in many ways but want to find a way to thrive in another area of their life.

Finally, she is a former Army, Non-Commissioned Officer, having honorably served 4 years Active Duty and 4 years Reserves as a Supply Sergeant.

Above all else professional, she is married to a wonderful husband and raising four amazing children and she could not be happier with their little brady bunch.

With all the hats she has worn and currently wears, she has always been motivated to give 110% of her efforts. She enjoys all the areas of her life and seeks to help others increase all the areas of their life.

Visit her at www.chattinwithcrystal.com